UNDERSTANDING EPILEPSY

Comprehensive Guide To Symptoms, Diagnosis, Treatment, And Management Strategies For Seizure Disorders

DR. LINCOLN WAYLON

DISCLAIMER

This book contains information that should only be used for educational and informational reasons; it is not meant to be used as a source of medical or psychological advice. The author's studies, life experiences, and expertise in the area of health and wellness served as the foundation for the content. It should not, however, be used in place of expert counsel, a diagnosis, or medical care.

Any queries you may have about a physical or mental health issue should always be directed toward the advice of a licensed healthcare provider or mental health specialist. With regard to the efficacy or outcomes of the methods or suggestions included in this book, the author and publisher make no representations or warranties.

Any information or methods in this book are used entirely at the reader's own risk and discretion. The material provided here may be used or misused, and neither the author nor the publisher will be held responsible for any results, losses, or negative impacts.

Keep in mind that everyone has different demands and reactions to health and wellness routines. Any health and wellness plans you implement must be customized to your particular circumstances, and you should speak with experts to make sure the plans meet your needs.

TABLE OF CONTENTS

ABOUT THE BOOK

The book Understanding Epilepsy is an essential resource for anyone seeking comprehensive knowledge about this complex neurological condition. It begins with a detailed overview of epilepsy, clarifying the definition, types of seizures, and how epilepsy differs from other neurological disorders. This foundational understanding is critical, as it dispels common myths and misconceptions, offering a clear picture of the prevalence and impact of epilepsy on individuals and society.

A crucial aspect of managing epilepsy involves accurate diagnosis. This book delves into the process of diagnosing epilepsy, highlighting the importance of medical history, symptoms, and diagnostic tests such as EEG, MRI, and CT scans.

It emphasizes the role of neurologists and epileptologists in navigating diagnostic challenges and underscores the importance of follow-up and monitoring to ensure effective management.

Managing seizure triggers is another vital topic covered, with a focus on identifying common triggers like stress and lack of sleep. The book offers practical advice on lifestyle adjustments, the significance of maintaining a seizure diary, and the role of diet, nutrition, and environmental modifications in minimizing triggers.

The treatment options for epilepsy are explored in depth, including an overview of antiepileptic drugs (AEDs), surgical interventions for refractory epilepsy, and newer treatments like vagus nerve stimulation and responsive neurostimulation. The book also discusses cognitive and behavioral therapies, as well as complementary and alternative treatments, providing a comprehensive guide to current and emerging therapeutic strategies.

Living with epilepsy presents unique challenges, which the book addresses with sensitivity and practical guidance. It covers managing daily life and activities, educational and workplace considerations, and the importance of emotional and psychological support. Building a support network and employing effective coping strategies are emphasized to help individuals navigate their daily lives.

For those affected by epilepsy at different life stages, the book provides tailored insights. It examines pediatric epilepsy, including the specific seizure types, diagnosis, and treatment considerations for children, and the impact on development, learning, and family dynamics. Similarly, it addresses adult-onset epilepsy, workplace management, social life, and reproductive health, along with the challenges of aging with epilepsy.

The book also equips readers with essential first aid knowledge, detailing the immediate response during a seizure, safety measures, and when to seek emergency help. Educating others about first aid is highlighted as a crucial aspect of managing epilepsy effectively.

In addition to practical advice, the book explores the latest advancements in epilepsy research, including emerging treatments, technologies, and clinical trials. It discusses how ongoing research impacts treatment options and the future directions in epilepsy care.

The book addresses common concerns and FAQs about living with epilepsy, including misconceptions, medication side effects, and social and legal issues. It provides valuable resources for further information and support, ensuring that readers are well-informed and empowered to manage epilepsy effectively.

CHAPTER ONE

OVERVIEW OF EPILEPSY

DEFINITION AND OVERVIEW

Epilepsy is a neurological disorder characterized by recurrent, unprovoked seizures that arise from abnormal electrical activity in the brain. These seizures can vary widely in their manifestation, from brief lapses in awareness to intense convulsions. The condition is chronic and can significantly affect a person's quality of life, impacting their ability to perform daily activities and maintain independence. Understanding epilepsy requires recognizing that it is not a single condition but a spectrum of disorders with diverse symptoms and triggers.

The diagnosis of epilepsy is typically made through a combination of medical history, neurological examination, and diagnostic tests such as EEGs (electroencephalograms) and MRI scans. An EEG records electrical activity in the brain and can help identify abnormal patterns associated with seizures.

It is crucial to differentiate between epilepsy and other conditions that may cause similar symptoms, such as syncope or transient ischemic attacks.

Management of epilepsy often involves medication to control seizures, lifestyle modifications to reduce triggers, and, in some cases, surgical interventions for refractory cases. While many people with epilepsy achieve good seizure control with treatment, ongoing medical care is essential to adapt therapy as needed and to address any side effects or complications.

TYPES OF SEIZURES

Seizures in epilepsy are categorized into two main types: focal (or partial) seizures and generalized seizures. Focal seizures originate in a specific area of the brain and can be further classified into focal onset aware seizures, where the person remains conscious, and focal onset impaired awareness seizures, where consciousness is affected. These seizures can vary from brief, subtle movements to more noticeable convulsions and may or may not spread to other parts of the brain.

Generalized seizures involve abnormal electrical activity across both hemispheres of the brain from the onset. They are further divided into several types, including tonic-clonic seizures, which are characterized by a combination of muscle stiffening and rhythmic jerking, and absence seizures, which cause brief lapses in consciousness. Other types include myoclonic seizures, which involve sudden muscle jerks, and atonic seizures, which result in a sudden loss of muscle tone.

Understanding the type of seizure a person experiences is crucial for effective management. Accurate seizure classification helps guide treatment decisions and informs strategies for seizure prevention and emergency response. In practice, this involves monitoring and documenting the nature of seizures, identifying triggers, and collaborating with healthcare providers to optimize treatment.

DISTINCTION FROM OTHER NEUROLOGICAL DISORDERS

Epilepsy is often confused with other neurological disorders due to overlapping symptoms, but it is essential to distinguish it from conditions such as migraines, transient ischemic attacks (TIAs), and psychogenic non-epileptic seizures (PNES). Migraines can sometimes involve auras that resemble seizures, but they are typically accompanied by headaches and are not associated with abnormal brain electrical activity.

TIAs, or mini-strokes, can cause transient symptoms similar to seizures, such as loss of consciousness or altered sensations. However, TIAs are due to temporary disruptions in blood flow to the brain and do not involve abnormal electrical activity. PNES, on the other hand, are episodes that mimic seizures but have psychological rather than neurological origins and require a different approach to diagnosis and treatment.

Accurate diagnosis involves a comprehensive evaluation, including neurological examinations, imaging studies, and EEGs, to differentiate epilepsy from other conditions. Understanding these distinctions helps ensure appropriate treatment and management strategies tailored to the specific underlying condition.

PREVALENCE AND IMPACT

Epilepsy affects approximately 1 in 100 people globally, making it one of the most common neurological disorders. The prevalence varies by age, with the highest rates observed in children and the elderly. The impact of epilepsy extends beyond the immediate medical effects, influencing various aspects of daily life, including employment, education, and social interactions.

People with epilepsy may face challenges such as stigma, discrimination, and barriers to accessing appropriate care and support. The unpredictability of seizures can also lead to difficulties in driving, working, and participating in recreational activities. Effective management and support systems are crucial in minimizing these impacts and improving overall quality of life.

Public awareness and education about epilepsy can help reduce stigma and improve the understanding of the condition. Initiatives aimed at increasing knowledge and empathy towards individuals with epilepsy can foster a more inclusive environment and support better outcomes for those affected.

COMMON MYTHS AND MISCONCEPTIONS

Epilepsy is often surrounded by myths and misconceptions that can hinder understanding and support.

A common myth is that epilepsy is a form of mental illness or that it is caused by personal weakness, which is not true. Epilepsy is a neurological disorder with identifiable causes and is not related to an individual's character or behavior.

Another misconception is that people with epilepsy should avoid physical activity or that they are incapable of leading normal lives. In reality, many individuals with epilepsy can engage in regular activities, including sports and work, with appropriate precautions and treatment. It is also a myth that seizures are always dangerous or uncontrollable; with proper management, many people experience significant seizure control.

Education and accurate information are key to dispelling these myths and improving the quality of life for individuals with epilepsy. Promoting awareness about the true nature of epilepsy can lead to better support, reduced stigma, and improved public understanding.

CHAPTER TWO

DIAGNOSING EPILEPSY

MEDICAL HISTORY AND SYMPTOMS

When diagnosing epilepsy, the first step involves gathering a detailed medical history. This includes understanding the patient's personal and family medical background, as well as the onset and nature of their seizures. Key aspects to note are the frequency, duration, and type of seizures experienced, along with any preceding symptoms such as aura or unusual sensations. The medical history should also encompass information about any head injuries, infections, or other conditions that might contribute to seizure activity. This comprehensive overview helps in differentiating epilepsy from other potential causes of seizures.

Symptoms reported by the patient are crucial in diagnosing epilepsy. Common symptoms include convulsions, loss of consciousness, and unusual movements or sensations. It is important to document whether seizures occur in clusters, if they are triggered by specific events, or if they happen spontaneously. Observations from family members or witnesses of the seizures can provide additional insights into the frequency and impact of the seizures on daily life. This detailed symptom profile guides the diagnostic process and helps in identifying the type of epilepsy.

In addition to personal symptoms, it is essential to consider the patient's response to any previous treatments or interventions. This includes reviewing past medications, their effectiveness, and any side effects experienced.

By understanding the patient's history and symptoms comprehensively, healthcare professionals can make informed decisions about further diagnostic testing and potential treatment options, paving the way for accurate diagnosis and effective management of epilepsy.

DIAGNOSTIC TESTS (EEG, MRI, CT)

Diagnostic tests are vital for confirming an epilepsy diagnosis and determining the underlying causes. Electroencephalography (EEG) is a key tool used to record electrical activity in the brain. It helps identify abnormal brain wave patterns characteristic of epilepsy.

During an EEG, electrodes are placed on the scalp to capture electrical signals. The results can show epileptiform discharges and aid in localizing the origin of the seizures, providing valuable information for diagnosis and treatment planning.

Magnetic Resonance Imaging (MRI) is used to visualize the brain's structure. It provides detailed images that can reveal structural abnormalities such as tumors, lesions, or malformations that might be causing seizures. MRI scans use strong magnetic fields and radio waves to create cross-sectional images of the brain. This test is non-invasive and helps in identifying structural changes that could contribute to seizure activity, aiding in both diagnosis and surgical planning if needed.

Computed Tomography (CT) scans are another imaging technique used to detect structural abnormalities in the brain. Unlike MRI, CT scans use X-rays to create detailed images and are often used in emergencies to quickly identify acute issues like bleeding or swelling. While less detailed than MRI, CT scans are useful for initial assessments and ruling out other potential causes of seizures. Together with EEG and MRI, CT scans contribute to a comprehensive diagnostic approach for epilepsy.

ROLE OF NEUROLOGISTS AND EPILEPTOLOGISTS

Neurologists and epileptologists play crucial roles in diagnosing and managing epilepsy. Neurologists are medical doctors specializing in disorders of the nervous system. They conduct initial evaluations, order diagnostic tests, and develop treatment plans for patients with epilepsy.

Their expertise covers a broad range of neurological conditions, allowing them to identify and treat various causes of seizures.

Epileptologists are neurologists with specialized training in epilepsy. They focus on the complex aspects of epilepsy diagnosis and treatment. They often handle cases that are difficult to manage or where standard treatments have failed. Epileptologists use advanced diagnostic techniques and are involved in research to explore new treatments and understand epilepsy better. Their expertise is particularly valuable for patients with drug-resistant epilepsy or those requiring surgical intervention.

Both neurologists and epileptologists work closely with other healthcare professionals, including nurses, psychologists, and social workers, to provide comprehensive care. They collaborate in creating individualized treatment plans, which may include medications, lifestyle adjustments, and, in some cases, surgical options.

Their combined efforts ensure that patients receive a thorough and effective approach to managing their epilepsy.

CHALLENGES IN DIAGNOSIS

Diagnosing epilepsy can be challenging due to the variability in seizure types and their presentations. Seizures can mimic other medical conditions such as fainting, migraines, or psychiatric disorders, making it difficult to distinguish them from non-epileptic events.

Accurate diagnosis requires careful differentiation between epileptic and non-epileptic seizures, which often involves a detailed history and multiple diagnostic tests.

Another challenge is that seizures may not always be captured during diagnostic tests. For instance, EEGs may miss seizure activity if the patient is not experiencing a seizure during the recording. This can lead to a false negative result and complicate the diagnosis. Long-term monitoring or repeated tests might be necessary to capture and analyze seizure activity accurately.

Patients with epilepsy may also experience variability in seizure patterns over time, making it challenging to pinpoint the exact nature and triggers of their seizures. This variability requires ongoing adjustments to the diagnostic approach and treatment plan, and continuous monitoring is essential to adapt to changes in seizure frequency and intensity.

FOLLOW-UP AND MONITORING

Follow-up and monitoring are essential components of epilepsy management. After an initial diagnosis, regular follow-up appointments are necessary to assess the effectiveness of the treatment plan and make any necessary adjustments. These appointments typically involve reviewing seizure frequency, medication side effects, and overall patient well-being.

Consistent monitoring helps ensure that treatment remains effective and that any emerging issues are promptly addressed.

Patients may undergo periodic EEGs and imaging studies to evaluate changes in their condition and to monitor the effects of treatment. These tests help track progress and detect any new abnormalities that may arise. Regular follow-up also provides an opportunity for healthcare professionals to educate patients about managing their condition, including lifestyle modifications and adherence to medication regimens.

In addition to clinical follow-ups, patients often benefit from support services such as counseling and educational resources. These services can help individuals and their families cope with the emotional and practical aspects of living with epilepsy. Effective follow-up and monitoring are crucial for optimizing treatment outcomes and improving the overall quality of life for patients with epilepsy.

CHAPTER THREE

MANAGING SEIZURE TRIGGERS

IDENTIFYING COMMON TRIGGERS

Recognizing the common triggers for seizures is crucial for managing epilepsy effectively. Stress, whether from emotional strain or physical pressure, is a prominent trigger that can lead to increased seizure activity. Identifying stressors in your life, such as work demands or personal issues, and finding ways to manage or reduce them can help mitigate seizure risks.

Similarly, lack of sleep is another significant trigger. Establishing a regular sleep routine and ensuring adequate rest each night can decrease the likelihood of seizures.

Other potential triggers include irregular medication adherence and substance use, such as alcohol or recreational drugs. It's important to follow prescribed medication schedules precisely and avoid substances known to trigger seizures. Tracking these factors in daily life can help in pinpointing specific triggers and managing them effectively. By recognizing and understanding these triggers, individuals can take proactive steps to minimize their impact on seizure activity.

LIFESTYLE ADJUSTMENTS TO AVOID TRIGGERS

Making strategic lifestyle adjustments is essential in managing epilepsy and reducing seizure frequency. Incorporating stress-reducing practices, such as regular exercise, meditation, or therapy, can help minimize the impact of stress on seizure activity. It's also important to establish a consistent daily routine, including regular sleep patterns and meal times, to support overall stability and health. Avoiding known triggers, such as excessive caffeine or late-night activities, can further contribute to better seizure control.

Additionally, engaging in supportive social activities and building a strong support network can help manage stress and provide emotional stability. Regular check-ins with healthcare professionals and adherence to prescribed treatments play a significant role in maintaining seizure control. Making these lifestyle changes not only helps in reducing seizures but also enhances overall well-being and quality of life.

IMPORTANCE OF A SEIZURE DIARY

Maintaining a seizure diary is a valuable tool for managing epilepsy and understanding seizure patterns. By documenting each seizure, including the date, time, duration, and any preceding factors, individuals can identify patterns or triggers that may be contributing to the seizures. This detailed record provides critical information for healthcare providers to adjust treatment plans and improve seizure management strategies.

A seizure diary also helps in tracking the effectiveness of medication and lifestyle adjustments. Observing changes over time allows for more informed discussions with healthcare professionals about treatment efficacy and necessary modifications. Consistent record-keeping can empower individuals to take an active role in their seizure management and contribute to more personalized and effective care.

ROLE OF DIET AND NUTRITION

Diet and nutrition play a significant role in managing epilepsy and supporting overall health. A balanced diet, rich in essential nutrients, can help stabilize energy levels and support neurological health. Certain dietary approaches, such as the ketogenic diet, may be recommended for individuals with epilepsy, as they have been shown to reduce seizure frequency in some cases. Consulting with a dietitian or healthcare provider to tailor dietary choices to individual needs can enhance seizure control.

Avoiding foods and substances that may trigger seizures, such as excessive sugar or artificial additives, is also important.

Regular meals and snacks can help maintain stable blood sugar levels, which may reduce the risk of seizures. Implementing a well-rounded, nutritious diet, and adhering to any specific dietary recommendations from healthcare providers, can contribute to effective epilepsy management and improved overall health.

ENVIRONMENTAL MODIFICATIONS

Making environmental modifications can help create a safer living space for individuals with epilepsy and reduce the risk of seizures. Implementing safety measures, such as removing sharp objects and installing safety rails, can minimize the risk of injury during a seizure. Adjusting the home environment to ensure it is seizure-friendly, such as using non-slip mats in the bathroom and ensuring adequate lighting, can further enhance safety.

Additionally, creating a seizure-friendly environment may involve modifying daily routines and activities to avoid potential triggers.

For instance, reducing exposure to flashing lights or loud noises, which can sometimes provoke seizures, can help in managing the condition. By making these practical changes, individuals can create a safer and more supportive environment, reducing the risk of seizures and enhancing overall quality of life.

CHAPTER FOUR

EPILEPSY TREATMENT OPTIONS
OVERVIEW OF ANTIEPILEPTIC DRUGS (AEDS)

Antiepileptic drugs (AEDs) are the cornerstone of epilepsy treatment, designed to control seizures and improve the quality of life for those with epilepsy. These medications work by stabilizing electrical activity in the brain. Common AEDs include carbamazepine, levetiracetam, and valproic acid, each targeting different types of seizures and brain activity disruptions. The choice of AED depends on the seizure type, the individual's overall health, and potential side effects. Monitoring and adjusting the dosage is crucial, as the goal is to balance seizure control with minimizing side effects.

Initiating AED treatment typically involves a trial-and-error approach to find the most effective medication with the fewest adverse effects. Doctors start with a standard dose and adjust based on the patient's response and tolerance. Regular follow-up appointments are essential to monitor the effectiveness of the treatment and make any necessary adjustments. Blood tests may be required to check drug levels and ensure they are within the therapeutic range, as well as to assess liver function and other parameters affected by the medication.

It is also vital for patients to be informed about the potential side effects and interactions of AEDs. Common side effects can include dizziness, fatigue, and gastrointestinal issues. Patients should be encouraged to report any unusual symptoms or side effects to their healthcare provider promptly. Adherence to the prescribed regimen is critical, as missing doses or stopping the medication abruptly can lead to an increase in seizure frequency or severity.

SURGICAL OPTIONS FOR REFRACTORY EPILEPSY

For individuals with refractory epilepsy, where seizures persist despite optimal medication, surgical options may be considered. One common surgical procedure is resection surgery, which involves removing the brain tissue where seizures originate. This approach is usually pursued after detailed pre-surgical evaluations, including imaging studies and EEG monitoring, to precisely identify the seizure focus. Success rates can be high, with many patients experiencing significant reductions in seizure frequency or even seizure freedom.

Another surgical approach is the implantation of a responsive neurostimulation (RNS) device, which detects abnormal electrical activity and delivers electrical pulses to prevent seizures. The device is implanted in the skull and connected to electrodes placed in or on the brain. This method is less invasive compared to resective surgery and is often chosen for patients who are not candidates for traditional surgery. Regular programming and adjustments of the RNS system are necessary to optimize its effectiveness.

Surgical interventions require a thorough evaluation by a specialized epilepsy center to assess suitability and potential risks. Post-surgery, patients may need rehabilitation and ongoing follow-up to monitor for complications and assess the success of the intervention. The goal is to achieve significant seizure reduction and improve overall quality of life while ensuring that the risks of surgery are outweighed by the potential benefits.

VAGUS NERVE STIMULATION AND RESPONSIVE NEUROSTIMULATION

Vagus nerve stimulation (VNS) is a therapeutic approach for epilepsy that involves implanting a small device under the skin of the chest, which sends regular electrical impulses to the vagus nerve in the neck. These impulses help modulate brain activity and can reduce the frequency and severity of seizures.

The device is programmable, allowing adjustments to the stimulation parameters based on the patient's needs.

VNS is typically considered when seizures are not well-controlled with medications and is often used in conjunction with other treatments.

Responsive neurostimulation (RNS) involves the implantation of a device that monitors brain activity and delivers electrical stimulation when abnormal activity is detected. This technology provides a more targeted approach by responding to the patient's specific seizure patterns. The RNS device is implanted in the skull, and electrodes are placed near the seizure focus. This method can be beneficial for patients with localized seizure origins and offers the advantage of real-time adjustment to prevent seizures.

Both VNS and RNS require regular follow-ups to adjust settings and evaluate their effectiveness. Patients may experience gradual improvements in seizure control, but results can vary. These treatments offer alternatives for those who do not respond well to medication alone and are a step forward in personalized epilepsy management, providing a more tailored approach to reducing seizures.

COGNITIVE AND BEHAVIORAL THERAPIES

Cognitive and behavioral therapies are adjunctive treatments for epilepsy that focus on managing the psychological and social aspects of living with the condition. Cognitive-behavioral therapy (CBT) is a common approach that helps individuals develop coping strategies for dealing with stress and anxiety related to their seizures. By addressing negative thought patterns and developing healthier coping mechanisms, CBT can improve overall mental well-being and quality of life.

Behavioral therapies often include techniques such as relaxation training and biofeedback, which help individuals manage the psychological impact of epilepsy. These therapies can be particularly useful for addressing issues like sleep disturbances, mood disorders, and stress, which can affect seizure frequency and severity.

Patients work with therapists to develop personalized strategies that fit their lifestyles and needs.

Incorporating cognitive and behavioral therapies into epilepsy treatment can provide comprehensive care, addressing both the neurological and psychological aspects of the condition. This holistic approach helps patients better manage their condition, improve adherence to other treatments, and enhance their overall quality of life. Collaboration with mental health professionals is essential to tailor these therapies to individual needs and ensure effective outcomes.

COMPLEMENTARY AND ALTERNATIVE TREATMENTS

Complementary and alternative treatments can be used alongside conventional epilepsy treatments to support overall well-being and potentially improve seizure control. These treatments include practices such as acupuncture, herbal supplements, and dietary changes. While some patients find these methods helpful, it is essential to consult with a healthcare provider before starting any complementary treatments, as they can interact with prescribed medications or have side effects.

Dietary approaches, such as the ketogenic diet, have shown promise in reducing seizures in some individuals. The ketogenic diet is a high-fat, low-carbohydrate diet that alters the body's metabolism to help control seizures. This diet must be followed under medical supervision to ensure nutritional balance and effectiveness. For some, dietary changes can be a beneficial adjunct to standard treatments.

Complementary therapies should be approached with caution and as part of a broader treatment plan. Patients must communicate openly with their healthcare team about any alternative treatments they are considering. This ensures that all aspects of their treatment are coordinated and that they receive the most comprehensive and effective care possible.

CHAPTER FIVE

LIVING WITH EPILEPSY

MANAGING DAILY LIFE AND ACTIVITIES

Living with epilepsy requires careful planning and management to ensure daily life runs smoothly. Establishing a consistent routine helps maintain stability and reduces the likelihood of seizure triggers. Create a daily schedule that includes regular sleep, meal times, and medication routines. Utilize tools like alarms or reminders for medication to ensure timely intake. Additionally, keeping a seizure diary can help track patterns and identify potential triggers, which is vital for managing the condition effectively.

Adapting activities and environments to accommodate epilepsy is crucial for safety and well-being. Engage in activities that are less likely to provoke seizures and modify those that pose risks. For instance, if swimming is a part of your routine, always ensure a safe environment with a supervising person. Also, make necessary adjustments in your home, such as installing grab bars in the bathroom or using non-slip mats, to prevent accidents during seizures.

Communicating openly with family members, friends, and caregivers about your condition is essential. Educate them on what to do in case of a seizure, including how to administer first aid if needed. This awareness not only helps them provide better support but also fosters a more understanding and accommodating environment.

EDUCATIONAL AND WORKPLACE CONSIDERATIONS

In educational settings, managing epilepsy involves working closely with teachers and school staff to ensure accommodations is in place. Inform the school about your condition and any special needs that may arise. This might include having extra time for assignments, access to a quiet place for rest, or modifications to physical activities that could trigger seizures. Regular meetings with school personnel can help keep everyone informed and prepared.

For workplace considerations, it's important to discuss your needs with your employer or human resources department. Employers are legally required to provide reasonable accommodations under disability laws, which may include adjusted work hours, changes in job responsibilities, or specialized equipment. Open communication about your condition and any potential challenges can help create a supportive work environment.

Maintaining a balance between managing your condition and pursuing educational or career goals is essential. Seek out resources and support services that can assist in overcoming barriers and achieving success.

EMOTIONAL AND PSYCHOLOGICAL SUPPORT

Living with epilepsy can impact mental health, making emotional and psychological support a key aspect of managing the condition. Engaging in therapy or counseling can help address feelings of anxiety, depression, or frustration that may arise. Professional support offers a safe space to explore and manage these emotions, contributing to overall well-being.

Self-help techniques such as mindfulness, relaxation exercises, and stress management can also be beneficial. Practices like deep breathing, meditation, and yoga can help reduce stress and anxiety, which might otherwise trigger seizures. Incorporating these practices into daily routines can improve emotional resilience and quality of life.

Building a positive mindset and focusing on personal strengths and achievements can aid in coping with the challenges of epilepsy. Setting realistic goals, celebrating successes, and maintaining a hopeful outlook are crucial for managing the psychological impact of the condition. Support groups and online communities can provide additional encouragement and shared experiences.

BUILDING A SUPPORT NETWORK

Creating a strong support network involves connecting with others who can provide understanding and assistance. Joining epilepsy support groups or online communities allows individuals to share experiences, advice, and encouragement. These connections can be invaluable for emotional support and practical tips for managing daily life with epilepsy.

Engaging with healthcare providers, such as neurologists and epilepsy specialists, is also an important aspect of building a support network.

Regular consultations with these professionals ensure ongoing medical support and guidance, helping to address any changes in your condition or treatment plan.

Family and friends play a crucial role in providing day-to-day support. Educate them about epilepsy, including seizure first aid and emergency procedures.

COPING STRATEGIES AND SELF-CARE

Effective coping strategies are essential for managing epilepsy and maintaining overall health. Develop a personalized plan that includes lifestyle modifications such as regular exercise, a balanced diet, and adequate sleep. These elements contribute to overall well-being and can help reduce seizure frequency and severity.

Self-care practices such as managing stress, avoiding known triggers, and adhering to prescribed treatments are vital. Techniques like setting realistic goals, using relaxation methods, and engaging in enjoyable activities can enhance quality of life. Consistently following these practices helps in managing both the physical and emotional aspects of epilepsy.

Regular medical check-ups and adherence to treatment plans are crucial for effective management.

CHAPTER SIX

EPILEPSY AND CHILDREN

PEDIATRIC SEIZURE TYPES AND CHARACTERISTICS

Epilepsy in children manifests through various seizure types, each with distinct characteristics. The most common types include generalized seizures, which affect both hemispheres of the brain, and focal seizures, which start in one area. Generalized seizures often involve loss of consciousness and can be further classified into tonic-clonic seizures, characterized by muscle rigidity and convulsions, and absence seizures, marked by brief lapses in consciousness. Focal seizures, on the other hand, may involve motor or sensory symptoms and can sometimes spread to become generalized. Recognizing these types is crucial for effective management and treatment.

The frequency, duration, and presentation of seizures can vary widely among children. Some seizures may last only a few seconds, while others can extend over several minutes. Symptoms during a seizure can include uncontrollable movements, unusual sensations, or altered awareness. Parents and caregivers need to observe and document these characteristics to aid in accurate diagnosis and treatment planning. Understanding the specific type of seizure helps healthcare providers tailor their approach and optimize outcomes for the child.

Seizure triggers and patterns are also important considerations. Triggers might include stress, lack of sleep, or specific foods.

Identifying these triggers can help in modifying the child's environment and lifestyle to minimize seizure occurrences. Additionally, keeping a seizure diary that records the frequency, duration, and potential triggers of seizures can provide valuable insights for healthcare professionals, leading to more effective management strategies and treatment adjustments.

DIAGNOSIS AND TREATMENT CONSIDERATIONS FOR CHILDREN

Accurate diagnosis of epilepsy in children involves a comprehensive evaluation, including medical history, neurological examinations, and diagnostic tests such as EEGs (electroencephalograms) and brain imaging. EEGs are crucial for identifying abnormal electrical brain activity associated with seizures, while brain scans like MRI or CT can reveal structural abnormalities. A thorough evaluation helps differentiate epilepsy from other conditions that might mimic seizure-like symptoms.

Treatment for pediatric epilepsy typically involves medication management, with antiepileptic drugs (AEDs) being the cornerstone of therapy. The choice of medication depends on the type of seizures, the child's age, and potential side effects. It's important to start with a single AED and adjust dosages as necessary, aiming for the most effective dose with the fewest side effects.

In some cases, if medication is not effective, additional treatments such as ketogenic diets, vagus nerve stimulation, or even surgical options might be considered.

Ongoing monitoring and follow-up are vital to ensure the effectiveness of the treatment regimen. Regular appointments with a neurologist are necessary to assess seizure control, manage side effects, and adjust treatments as needed. Additionally, maintaining open communication with the healthcare team and reporting any changes in seizure frequency or new symptoms promptly can help in optimizing the treatment plan and improving the child's quality of life.

IMPACT ON DEVELOPMENT AND LEARNING

Epilepsy can have a significant impact on a child's developmental milestones and learning abilities. Seizures, particularly if frequent or severe, may interfere with cognitive functions, leading to challenges in attention, memory, and processing speed. Children with uncontrolled seizures might experience delays in reaching developmental milestones and may struggle with academic performance due to difficulties in concentrating and retaining information.

Educational interventions and accommodations can play a crucial role in supporting children with epilepsy. It is beneficial to work with teachers and school counselors to create an individualized education plan (IEP) that addresses specific learning needs and includes strategies to manage seizure-related disruptions. Regular communication between parents, educators, and healthcare providers ensures that the child's educational needs are met and that appropriate supports are in place.

In addition to cognitive and academic effects, children with epilepsy might face social challenges. Peer relationships can be impacted by the stigma associated with epilepsy or the visible effects of seizures. Providing social support and fostering an inclusive environment can help mitigate these challenges. Encouraging positive social interactions and addressing any concerns or misconceptions about epilepsy can contribute to a more supportive and understanding social environment for the child.

SCHOOL AND SOCIAL SUPPORT

Schools play a vital role in supporting children with epilepsy by providing a safe and accommodating learning environment. Teachers and school staff need to be educated about the child's condition, including recognizing seizure types, understanding emergency protocols, and knowing how to administer any necessary medications. Establishing a clear action plan for managing seizures at school, including who to contact and what steps to take during a seizure, is crucial for ensuring the child's safety and well-being.

Social support extends beyond the school setting and involves creating a supportive network for the child. Peer support programs, counseling services, and support groups can help children with epilepsy feel understood and less isolated.

Engaging in activities that build confidence and promote social skills can also be beneficial. Encouraging participation in extracurricular activities, while being mindful of the child's condition and potential triggers, can help foster a sense of normalcy and inclusion.

Parents and caregivers should advocate for their child's needs within the school and community. Building strong relationships with educators, participating in school meetings, and educating others about epilepsy can help ensure that the child receives the necessary accommodations and support. Effective communication and collaboration between home, school, and community resources contribute to a more supportive environment and better overall outcomes for the child.

FAMILY DYNAMICS AND COPING

Epilepsy can significantly affect family dynamics, as parents and siblings adjust to the demands of managing a chronic condition.

Families may experience a range of emotions, including stress, anxiety, and frustration, as they navigate the challenges of caring for a child with epilepsy. Families need to seek support and access resources that can provide practical advice and emotional assistance.

Family coping strategies can include joining support groups, where parents and caregivers can share experiences and gain insights from others in similar situations. Counseling and therapy can also be beneficial in helping family members process their emotions and develop effective coping mechanisms.

Balancing the needs of a child with epilepsy and maintaining family routines and relationships can be challenging. Establishing a structured routine that includes medical appointments, medication schedules, and family activities can help manage the condition while preserving family cohesion.

CHAPTER SEVEN

EPILEPSY AND ADULTS

ADULT-ONSET EPILEPSY

Adult-onset epilepsy is diagnosed when an individual begins experiencing seizures for the first time in adulthood, rather than in childhood. The condition can be triggered by various factors such as brain injuries, strokes, or infections. Diagnosing adult-onset epilepsy involves a comprehensive evaluation, including a detailed medical history, neurological examination, and diagnostic tests such as electroencephalograms (EEGs) and brain imaging. Identifying the underlying cause is crucial, as it may influence the treatment approach.

Management of adult-onset epilepsy typically includes anti-seizure medications tailored to the individual's specific type of epilepsy and seizure frequency. Lifestyle modifications, such as maintaining a regular sleep schedule and avoiding known seizure triggers, are also important. Regular follow-ups with a neurologist help in monitoring the effectiveness of the treatment and making any necessary adjustments to the medication regimen.

In addition to medical management, individuals with adult-onset epilepsy should be educated about the condition and its impact on daily life. Support groups and counseling can provide emotional support and practical advice. Awareness and understanding of the condition by family, friends, and colleagues are essential for managing the challenges that come with adult-onset epilepsy.

MANAGING EPILEPSY IN THE WORKPLACE

Managing epilepsy in the workplace requires careful planning and communication to ensure a supportive environment. Employees with epilepsy should work with their employer to create an appropriate accommodation plan that may include adjustments to the work environment, such as flexible scheduling or modified duties.

Clear communication about the nature of the condition and potential needs is key to fostering an inclusive and understanding workplace.

Employers should be educated about epilepsy to prevent misunderstandings and ensure a safe working environment. Training programs can help colleagues recognize seizure symptoms and respond appropriately in case of an emergency.

Employers are legally required to provide reasonable accommodations under the Americans with Disabilities Act (ADA), which includes adjusting work conditions and providing necessary support.

Employees with epilepsy can benefit from developing a personalized action plan outlining seizure management strategies and emergency procedures. This plan should be shared with supervisors and key personnel to ensure everyone is prepared to assist if a seizure occurs.

Regular check-ins with human resources and healthcare providers can help address any ongoing concerns and make necessary adjustments to the work environment.

RELATIONSHIPS AND SOCIAL LIFE

Epilepsy can impact relationships and social interactions, often leading to challenges in communication and social integration. It is important for individuals with epilepsy to openly discuss their condition with partners, family, and friends to foster understanding and support.

Education about epilepsy can help alleviate misconceptions and reduce stigma, making it easier for loved ones to offer appropriate support.

Maintaining a healthy social life involves finding a balance between managing the condition and participating in activities. Joining support groups or engaging in community activities can provide opportunities for social interaction with others who have similar experiences. Developing coping strategies, such as stress management techniques and setting realistic social goals, can also help in maintaining a fulfilling social life.

Building strong and supportive relationships is crucial for emotional well-being. Individuals with epilepsy should seek out understanding and empathetic friends and partners who are willing to learn about the condition and its effects. Effective communication and mutual support play a significant role in managing the challenges that epilepsy can pose in personal relationships.

HANDLING PREGNANCY AND REPRODUCTIVE HEALTH

Managing epilepsy during pregnancy requires careful planning and coordination between the obstetrician and neurologist. Antiepileptic medications must be reviewed and adjusted as needed to minimize risks to both the mother and the developing baby. Regular prenatal care, including monitoring for potential complications and ensuring optimal seizure control, is essential for a healthy pregnancy.

Women with epilepsy should be informed about the potential effects of pregnancy on their condition, as hormonal changes and increased physical stress can influence seizure activity.

It is also important to discuss contraceptive options and family planning with a healthcare provider to make informed decisions regarding reproductive health. Preconception counseling can help address any concerns and develop a comprehensive care plan.

Postpartum care involves monitoring for any changes in seizure frequency or medication needs. Breastfeeding can be safely managed with appropriate medication adjustments, but it is important to consult with healthcare providers about potential risks and benefits. Overall, a collaborative approach with healthcare professionals can help ensure a healthy pregnancy and effective management of epilepsy.

AGING WITH EPILEPSY

Aging with epilepsy presents unique challenges that require careful management of both the condition and age-related health issues. As individuals with epilepsy age, they may experience changes in seizure patterns and an increased risk of coexisting medical conditions, such as cardiovascular disease or cognitive decline. Regular medical evaluations are crucial for adjusting treatment plans and addressing any new health concerns.

Older adults with epilepsy may need to modify their seizure management strategies to accommodate changes in metabolism and medication interactions. It is important to monitor for potential side effects of antiepileptic drugs, which may be more pronounced in older individuals.

Adapting lifestyle factors, such as maintaining physical activity and managing stress, can also contribute to better seizure control and overall health.

Support systems play a vital role in aging with epilepsy. Family members, caregivers, and healthcare providers should work together to ensure that the individual's needs are met and that they receive appropriate support. Access to community resources and support groups for older adults with epilepsy can provide valuable assistance in managing the challenges of aging with this condition.

CHAPTER EIGHT

FIRST AID FOR SEIZURES

IMMEDIATE RESPONSE DURING A SEIZURE

When someone is having a seizure, it's crucial to stay calm and ensure their safety. Begin by gently guiding them away from potential hazards such as sharp objects or hard surfaces. If possible, cushion their head with a soft item like a folded jacket or a pillow to prevent head injury. Avoid restraining their movements or putting anything in their mouth, as this can cause more harm than good. Keep track of the duration of the seizure, as this information will be helpful to medical professionals later.

Observe the person closely to ensure they do not fall or hurt themselves during the episode. If they are lying on the ground, place them in a recovery position on their side once the convulsions have stopped. This helps to keep their airway clear and allows any fluids to drain from their mouth, reducing the risk of choking. Avoid offering food or drink immediately after the seizure, as they may still be disoriented or have difficulty swallowing.

Remain with the person until they regain full consciousness and are alert. Offer reassurance and comfort as they may be confused or disoriented. If the seizure lasts more than five minutes, or if another seizure follows immediately, seek emergency medical assistance right away. Knowing how to respond quickly and effectively can significantly impact the safety and recovery of someone experiencing a seizure.

WHAT TO DO AND WHAT NOT TO DO

During a seizure, it is essential to focus on what actions will best ensure the person's safety. Do stay with them throughout the event and make a note of how long it lasts. Do keep the area around them clear of potential dangers. Do not try to hold the person down or restrain their movements, as this can lead to injuries or worsen the seizure.

Do not attempt to put anything in their mouth; this can cause choking or damage to the person's teeth and gums.

Avoid giving the person any food or drink until they are fully alert and able to swallow safely. It is important not to engage in any unnecessary conversation or make judgments about the situation. Do not leave the person alone until they have completely recovered and are fully conscious. Ensuring these dos and don'ts are followed can help prevent further complications and ensure the individual's safety during a seizure.

Educating yourself and others about these critical actions can make a significant difference in managing seizure episodes effectively. By understanding what to do and what to avoid, you can provide better support and reduce the risk of harm during such emergencies. Always stay informed and prepared to handle such situations with care and knowledge.

SAFETY MEASURES FOR SEIZURE EPISODES

Implementing safety measures during a seizure can greatly reduce the risk of injury. Ensure that the environment is safe by removing sharp objects, hard furniture, or anything that could potentially harm the individual if they fall. If the person is in bed, place a padded cushion or soft material around them to minimize injury from sudden movements. Securing the immediate area helps prevent accidents and provides a safer environment during the seizure.

Be mindful of the person's comfort and safety post-seizure. After the episode, help them into a comfortable and safe position, such as lying on their side. This position helps keep their airway clear and allows them to breathe more easily. Ensure the area around them remains free of obstacles that could pose risks if they are unsteady or confused upon waking. Implementing these safety measures helps in managing the situation effectively and can prevent further complications.

Educating family members, caregivers, and others about these safety measures is crucial. Everyone involved should understand how to create a safe environment and what steps to take before, during, and after a seizure. By promoting awareness and preparedness, you contribute to a safer space for those who may experience seizures.

WHEN TO SEEK EMERGENCY HELP

Recognizing when to seek emergency help is vital in managing seizures effectively. If a seizure lasts more than five minutes or if another seizure follows immediately, you should call for medical assistance right away.

Immediate medical attention is necessary to address prolonged or consecutive seizures, which can indicate a serious underlying issue or pose increased health risks.

Emergency help is also required if the person is injured during the seizure, has difficulty breathing, or shows signs of a possible medical complication. Additionally, if the person has never had a seizure before, or if this is a first-time occurrence, seeking prompt medical evaluation is important to determine the cause and appropriate treatment.

Lastly, if the individual does not regain consciousness or appears to be in distress after the seizure, it's essential to contact emergency services. Professional medical assessment and intervention are critical in these cases to ensure the person receives the appropriate care and support.

EDUCATING OTHERS ABOUT FIRST AID

Educating others about first aid for seizures is crucial in creating a supportive and prepared environment. Begin by explaining the basics of what a seizure is and how it may appear.

Provide clear instructions on how to respond, including how to keep the person safe, what actions to avoid, and when to seek emergency help.

Ensuring that everyone involved is aware of these steps can greatly improve the handling of seizure situations.

Host training sessions or provide written materials that detail first aid procedures for seizures. These resources should cover immediate responses, safety measures, and emergency protocols. Engaging with community groups, schools, and workplaces to disseminate this information can help build a network of knowledgeable individuals who can assist in a seizure episode.

Encourage regular updates and refreshers on first aid practices for seizures, as understanding and preparedness can make a significant difference in emergencies. By fostering a culture of education and awareness, you contribute to better outcomes for individuals experiencing seizures and ensure a more informed response from those around them.

CHAPTER NINE

EPILEPSY RESEARCH AND ADVANCES

LATEST ADVANCEMENTS IN EPILEPSY RESEARCH

Recent advancements in epilepsy research have significantly enhanced our understanding of the condition. Breakthroughs in neuroimaging, such as high-resolution MRI and PET scans, allow researchers to better visualize brain abnormalities associated with epilepsy. These imaging techniques are crucial in identifying the exact locations of seizures, leading to more precise diagnostic and surgical interventions. Additionally, genetic research has uncovered specific gene mutations linked to various forms of epilepsy, paving the way for personalized medicine approaches that target these genetic abnormalities directly.

Another exciting development is the use of advanced computational models and artificial intelligence to analyze seizure patterns and predict epilepsy onset.

Machine learning algorithms can process vast amounts of data from EEGs and other monitoring devices, offering new insights into seizure triggers and responses to treatment. These models help in tailoring individualized treatment plans and improving overall patient outcomes by predicting seizure occurrences with greater accuracy.

Furthermore, research into neurostimulation techniques, such as responsive neurostimulation (RNS) and deep brain stimulation (DBS), has shown promising results. These methods involve implanting devices that detect and respond to seizure activity in real time, thereby reducing the frequency and severity of seizures. The ongoing refinement and testing of these technologies are expected to provide more effective and targeted treatment options for individuals with epilepsy.

EMERGING TREATMENTS AND TECHNOLOGIES

Emerging treatments and technologies for epilepsy are transforming patient care by offering new therapeutic options. One notable advancement is the development of novel antiepileptic drugs (AEDs) with improved efficacy and fewer side effects compared to traditional medications. These new drugs are designed to target specific neurotransmitter systems and ion channels involved in seizure activity, providing more effective seizure control for patients who do not respond well to conventional treatments.

In addition to pharmacological advances, non-drug therapies such as ketogenic diets and vagus nerve stimulation (VNS) are gaining traction.

The ketogenic diet, a high-fat, low-carbohydrate regimen, has been shown to reduce seizure frequency in some patients, particularly those with drug-resistant epilepsy. VNS, which involves implanting a device that stimulates the vagus nerve, offers a complementary approach for managing seizures and improving overall quality of life.

Wearable technologies and mobile apps are also making significant strides in epilepsy management.

These tools allow patients to monitor their seizure activity, medication adherence, and triggers in real time. Data collected from these devices can be shared with healthcare providers to adjust treatment plans and track progress, leading to more personalized and effective management strategies.

CLINICAL TRIALS AND PARTICIPATION

Participating in clinical trials is a critical component of advancing epilepsy research and treatment. Clinical trials test new drugs, devices, or therapies to determine their safety and effectiveness. Patients who enroll in these trials contribute to the development of innovative treatments that may eventually benefit a broader population. Participation involves careful screening to ensure eligibility, followed by regular monitoring and assessments to track the effects of the experimental intervention.

For those considering participation, it's essential to understand the trial's purpose, potential benefits, and risks.

Clinical trials are conducted in phases, starting with small groups of participants to assess safety before expanding to larger populations to evaluate efficacy. Participants may receive the new treatment, a placebo, or the standard of care, depending on the trial's design. Clear communication with the research team and understanding the trial's requirements and procedures are crucial for making an informed decision.

Moreover, the results from clinical trials provide valuable data that drive future research directions and treatment innovations. By participating, individuals contribute to a collective effort to improve epilepsy care and treatment options, potentially leading to breakthroughs that can transform the management of the condition on a global scale.

FUTURE DIRECTIONS IN EPILEPSY CARE

The future of epilepsy care holds exciting possibilities driven by ongoing research and technological advancements.

One promising direction is the integration of precision medicine approaches, where treatments are tailored to the individual's genetic and physiological characteristics. This personalized approach aims to optimize treatment effectiveness and minimize adverse effects by targeting the underlying causes of epilepsy more precisely.

Advancements in neurotechnology, such as brain-computer interfaces and next-generation neurostimulation devices, are expected to revolutionize epilepsy management. These technologies could offer new ways to monitor brain activity, deliver targeted treatments, and even potentially modulate brain function to prevent seizures before they occur. Research is also exploring the use of advanced imaging and electrophysiological techniques to better understand and predict seizure dynamics, leading to more effective interventions.

Additionally, there is a growing emphasis on improving patient quality of life through holistic care approaches.

This includes addressing comorbid conditions, providing psychological support, and integrating lifestyle modifications into treatment plans. Future epilepsy care models are likely to focus on comprehensive management strategies that consider the overall well-being of the patient, not just the control of seizures.

HOW RESEARCH IMPACTS TREATMENT OPTIONS

Research plays a pivotal role in shaping the treatment options available for epilepsy. Innovations and discoveries from ongoing studies lead to the development of new medications, therapies, and diagnostic tools. For instance, research into the mechanisms of seizure generation and propagation has led to the creation of targeted drugs that address specific aspects of epileptic activity, improving treatment outcomes for patients who have not responded well to standard medications.

Clinical trials and research studies also provide evidence-based data that guide clinical practice and treatment guidelines. As new findings emerge, they inform updates to treatment protocols and recommendations, ensuring that patients have access to the most current and effective therapies. Research findings can also highlight gaps in existing treatments, prompting further investigation and the development of novel approaches to address unmet needs.

Furthermore, patient participation in research contributes to a better understanding of how different treatments work in diverse populations. This real-world data helps refine treatment strategies and develop personalized approaches to care, ultimately improving the overall effectiveness and safety of epilepsy management. By bridging the gap between laboratory research and clinical application, ongoing studies continue to enhance treatment options and patient outcomes in epilepsy care.

CHAPTER TEN

COMMON CONCERNS AND FAQS

ADDRESSING COMMON MISCONCEPTIONS

Epilepsy is often surrounded by myths that can lead to misunderstanding and stigma. One prevalent misconception is that people with epilepsy are incapable of leading normal lives, which is far from the truth. Many individuals with epilepsy successfully manage their condition with appropriate treatment and lifestyle adjustments.

It's essential to understand that epilepsy does not define a person's abilities or potential and that many people with epilepsy lead fulfilling careers and maintain healthy relationships.

Another misconception is that seizures always result in a loss of consciousness or convulsions. In reality, epilepsy encompasses a wide range of seizure types, including those that cause brief lapses in awareness or subtle changes in sensation.

Understanding the diversity of seizures helps in recognizing that not all seizures are dramatic or noticeable, which is crucial for supporting someone with epilepsy appropriately.

Lastly, there is a belief that epilepsy is a mental illness caused by psychological issues. This is incorrect, as epilepsy is a neurological disorder resulting from abnormal electrical activity in the brain. Educating oneself and others about the neurological basis of epilepsy can help in reducing stigma and fostering a more accurate understanding of the condition.

FAQS ABOUT LIVING WITH EPILEPSY

Living with epilepsy often raises practical questions about day-to-day management. One common query is how to handle seizures in public settings. Individuals with epilepsy need to have a clear plan for managing seizures when they occur, including informing friends and family about appropriate responses, such as keeping the person safe and ensuring they have a medical ID. It's also useful to discuss seizure management strategies with a healthcare provider to tailor them to individual needs.

Another frequently asked question is about lifestyle adjustments. Many people with epilepsy wonder about the impact of diet, sleep, and exercise on their condition. Maintaining a regular sleep schedule, avoiding known seizure triggers like flashing lights or stress, and following a balanced diet can be beneficial. It's important to consult with a healthcare provider to develop a personalized plan that takes into account individual triggers and health goals.

People often also ask about driving and other activities. The rules about driving vary by location, but generally, individuals with epilepsy must be seizure-free for a specific period before they are legally allowed to drive. It's crucial to adhere to these regulations for safety and to consult with a healthcare provider about when it's appropriate to resume activities like driving or participating in sports.

CONCERNS ABOUT MEDICATIONS AND SIDE EFFECTS

Epilepsy treatment typically involves antiepileptic drugs (AEDs), and managing their side effects can be a significant concern. One common issue is the range of side effects, which can include fatigue, dizziness, and weight changes. Individuals need to communicate with their healthcare providers about any side effects they experience so that adjustments can be made to the medication or dosage. Regular follow-ups and open discussions with a doctor can help in managing these effects effectively.

Another concern is the effectiveness of different medications. Some people may need to try several AEDs to find the one that best controls their seizures with minimal side effects. This process can involve a trial-and-error approach, and patients must stay patient and persistent while working with their healthcare provider to find the most effective treatment regimen.

Additionally, many individuals worry about the long-term use of medications and their impact on overall health. Long-term medication use may lead to concerns about potential effects on bone health, liver function, or other aspects of physical well-being. Regular medical check-ups and monitoring can help in identifying and addressing any long-term effects early, ensuring ongoing health and well-being.

QUESTIONS ABOUT SOCIAL AND LEGAL ISSUES

Epilepsy can present various social and legal challenges that individuals may need to navigate. One common concern is discrimination or misunderstanding in the workplace. Individuals need to understand their rights under disability and employment laws, which can provide protection against discrimination and ensure reasonable accommodations are made.

Advocating for oneself and seeking support from epilepsy organizations can help in addressing these challenges effectively.

Another social concern involves stigma and the social isolation that may come with having epilepsy. People may face misconceptions or fear from others, leading to feelings of isolation. Engaging in support groups or community organizations can provide emotional support and practical advice on how to manage these social challenges and connect with others who understand the experience.

Legal issues related to epilepsy also include managing medical insurance and coverage for treatments. Navigating insurance policies can be complex, and understanding what is covered and how to appeal denied claims is crucial. Consulting with a legal advisor or an epilepsy support organization can guide managing insurance issues and ensuring access to necessary treatments and services.

RESOURCES FOR FURTHER INFORMATION AND SUPPORT

For individuals seeking more information and support about epilepsy, numerous resources are available. National epilepsy organizations provide valuable information, support groups, and advocacy services. Websites of organizations like the Epilepsy Foundation or the International League Against Epilepsy offer comprehensive resources, including educational materials, treatment guidelines, and community forums.

Local support groups and epilepsy centers can also offer personalized assistance and connect individuals with others facing similar challenges. These groups often provide opportunities for education, support, and advocacy, as well as practical advice on managing everyday issues related to epilepsy.

Additionally, healthcare providers can be a crucial resource for information and support. Regular consultations with neurologists or epilepsy specialists can provide up-to-date knowledge on treatment options, seizure management strategies, and coping techniques.